You Need to Heal Yourself

Some Ways to Make You in a Good Health

Table of Contents

Abstract

Healing yourself speaks to some of the greatest health authorities today. They talk directly to the viewer and break down the key steps that affect your health. These include: food and nutrition. Emotional and environmental stress. Mind energy; self-education hopes; love - plus the practical steps you can take to start restoring your health. This wall-to-wall information does not address the critical problems necessary to deal with, maintain, or restore your health.

Here are some ways that will help you to heal yourself in simple and easy path. Just follow these advices and I am sure you will find the good results in your body, your life, and your environment.

Introduction

I'm very tired of all the challenges of life! Are You? This world is poisonous and sick. I hate watching news or reading the newspaper or even interacting with my neighbors. I do not want to appear hostile to society. I really love people. But this world has made us cold and cruel.

Most of us reach painkillers at the first signs of headache or cold, but the art of self-healing is more popular among alternative medicine

The result is a community of unhappy people. More than 50% of all marriages end with divorce. More than 50% of all young people do not even believe in marriage. We need to go back to the days when it was easy to talk to outsiders and it was not natural to be polite.

Back to the days where people really believe in love and looking for their neighbors. We need to start loving ourselves again. Each of us needs the change we want to see in the world. We need to treat ourselves and start loving ourselves again.

Happy people are successful people. This is simply because happiness makes it easy to keep motivated to reach your goals. Your thoughts have a very significant impact on the life-led and quality relationships that you will enjoy with family and friends and others are important. So that some thoughts that our ideas and beliefs can have a stronger effect on our health than modern medicine. Consider these examples:

- Some human died just after being diagnosed with dangers illness like cancer or heart attack although it may be a diagnostic error.

- Many women who are desperate to have a child will start with real pregnancy symptoms such as cravings and increased breast size, despite the fact that they are not pregnant.

- Many people feel better after taking placebo even on chronic diseases such as depression and high cholesterol.

However, it has been scientifically proven that you can improve your health, your career and your relationships simply by improving your way of thinking about yourself and the world around you. It is important to learn from the challenges and changes we face that will give us a motive to resist the negative changes in our lives. This is much cheaper than paying encounters with a therapist or paying a divorce attorney.

The right food, the right exercise, the right medications, the right relationships - all of these things can help support the healing process, but only if you do it intentionally. Your deliberate conscious mind (which is separate from the subconscious and your nervous system, though connected to it) is the key to healing yourself.

Therapists often divide the physical, mental and spiritual parts of our nature to make healing simpler. Remember true healing, as it is about perfection, must always balance the mind, body and soul in the result. While the process of healing may begin with a simple beginning of the process of fixing one part of our nature: the process of healing large will always become a fabric of actions that combine elements of physical, mental and spiritual elements in one's life.

Healing yourself is not about going back to the previous situation from where you were before! To do that actually limits then helps to promote decay in the person's spirit. It is important that healing technology is always part of a more comprehensive growth process, rather than one simple constant procedure.

This book aims to help you heal yourself from all scars and the impact of all the negative surrounding them. As a result of healing, yourself must take into account how you work with the challenges in life.I guarantee that learning to rid yourself of the pain of this world will greatly improve your quality of life from this point forward.

Chapter 1 - who are you?

"To know thyself is the beginning of wisdom." –

Socrates

Knowing who you are is very important to treat yourself side. How can you avoid the difficulties of life if you simply float in life without a clear sense of what it represents, and refuses to bear?

Ask yourself what makes me happy?

What thinks I love to do?

Also think of the doctor which become a doctor because his father decided that. What about the boy chosen by his mother to be an engineer just because the happiness of his mother?

Why are you afraid to make your choice with your full will and do what you want to do and not what you should do?

The problem can be explained in the old proverb which points out that if we do not know where we are going, any way would be the right way. Better yet, "if we do not stand for something, we will drop anything." In other words, if we do not understand ourselves, it includes our hopes, our dreams and our aspirations, it will be easy for anyone to push us to a regrettable decision for the rest of our lives. Living in a regrettable choice, especially if you have to face its consequences on a daily basis, will be one of the most difficult things I have had to do. Living with the burden of these options is part of the reason why many people feel bitterness and cruelty. This is not the way you want to move through your life.

Is there a reason of your existence look for it in your heart? Your heart is the resource of happiness.

When we take the time to understand who we really are, the complexities of our personalities, we will have the keys to unlock our real capabilities. You cannot become yourself better if you do not know what it entails. When you understand yourself, you are more likely to end up choosing a career that you love. It is easy to be driven with enthusiasm to achieve great things when pursuing a career you love.

In addition, when you are at the top of your game, you will be looking for the kind of partners and friends who will make you happy and thus come out with the best of you. They will understand your thinking and may think the same way you think. These are people who will not laugh at your dreams or feel jealous of your success. Being surrounded by loving and supportive people will make you more pleasant and happy and dare to say a more successful person.

Do people around me understand me and understand my thoughts and do not mock my dreams?

Individuals who have a deep understanding of themselves are often more decisive and optimistic. This is because these individuals are in full control over their life choices and their choice well. They are more likely to see opportunities where others see setbacks. It also takes far less effort to be productive when you enjoy what you do. In addition, the fact that you enjoy your career will give you a competitive advantage and will not depend on the praise of others for motivation. Your satisfaction with good work will keep you moving forward.

I know that this may seem ideal, as our choices do not depend on the wishes of our family, and we are all strong enough not to be pressured into making a decision. But believe me, knowing yourself and your true understanding will open the doors to opportunities you never saw. It will be easier for you to cope with the pressure around you when you know without a doubt what the right decision will be for you. I do not encourage you to ignore your responsibilities to support your family. I encourage you to understand your identity and to be honest with who you are at all times. You will be happier as a result, and much easier to love, when you do not carry heavy weight for a bad decision throughout the rest of your life.

But how can I get to know myself? This is not impossible. You can start with some objective assessment. This does not mean just asking people about what they are thinking. Your interaction with them, whether negative or positive, will prevent them from being as objective as you need them. The best choice is to use a respectable personal test. There are many personal tests like Myers-Briggs have gained popularity lately because their results can be used to determine which environment works best in, and even how they interact with people around you. Plus whether you like the results or not tends to be surprisingly accurate.

Proficiency tests are another wonderful option. They are designed to help you better understand your skill set and how you can use these skills to identify the right occupation. It is not too late to start a career you can love.

Once you have a carefully thought out plan that allows you to take care of your responsibilities and still venturing into a field you love, go to it. There may be a case of money tight and you are already have a lack of time and may not be able to move now. But I encourage you to continue to prepare yourself. Keep learning all you can about the profession online or from people around you. This way, if you have the opportunity, you will be in a position to take it.

When you take the time to get to know yourself, you may find some hidden scars that may have been hidden deep within your personality. Unfortunately, these scars penetrated yourself while interacting with those around you. These scars may have made you too weak to express your feeling of cold and feeling comfortable with others' feelings. Now you can see yourself clearly and become the best copy for yourself. Love yourself. Above all, be honest with yourself. Knowing your limits is another important skill to master in order to navigate through this crazy world successfully.

The Benefits of Self-Knowledge:

> ➤ Happiness. You will be happier when you can express who you are. Expressing your desires, moreover, will make it more likely that you get what you want.

➤ Less inner conflict. When your outside actions are in accordance with your inside feelings and values, you will experience less inner conflict.

➤ Better decision-making. When you know yourself, you are able to make better choices about everything, from small decisions like which sweater you'll buy to big decisions like which partner you'll spend your life with. You'll have guidelines you can apply to solve life's varied problems.

➤ Self-control. When you know yourself, you understand what motivates you to resist bad habits and develop good ones. You'll have the insight to know which values and goals activate your willpower.

➤ Resistance to social pressure. When you are grounded in your values and preferences, you are less likely to say "yes" when you want to say "no."

➢ Tolerance and understanding of others. Your awareness of your own foibles and struggles can help you empathize with others.

➢ Vitality and pleasure: Being who you truly are helps you feel more alive and makes your experience of life richer, larger, and more exciting.

Chapter two what is your position?

"Humility is the road to success"

A key aspect of the Myers-Briggs Personality test results is the section that identifies your strengths and weaknesses. Many of the mistakes we made and the problems we face could have been avoided if we were more familiar with our minors. Just think of weightlifting eager to try to raise a lot, very soon. What do you think will happen? Any sane individual will realize that weight lifting will hurt himself. Some will say that this clarification encourages us to limit ourselves, and if we do, and stop pushing ourselves, we will never know our real potential.

There is no limit to what you can achieve if you put your mind on it, and sometimes you will never know your strength except you try it. But you need to make sure that reason and logic prevail when you reach your goals. If you never lift 100 pounds, starting 20 pounds today might be a better idea. There's nothing wrong with thinking a lot, but I encourage you to start working small. I encourage you to be modest in your expectations.

Modesty will not only help you avoid unrealistic expectations, it will also help you set realistic time frames to achieve your goals. Many people become frustrated when they reach a certain age and do not achieve a certain goal.

Choosing a career in a field you love will help you stay motivated and become successful. This theory appears in the lives of each of these men. Their success was due to their passion for something they loved.

A modest approach to life will help you avoid comparing your achievements with those of others. Some people hit the ball from the park on the first try, and there are others who have to work their way up the ladder. Some will get married right out of college, while others should wait a few years before some frogs before finding the right person. Do not expect your life to be different. No matter what you want to achieve, you have to work harder than ever and you may have to wait longer than expected.

The beautiful kind of humility goes beyond success. This is the quality that will help you to stop biting more than you can chew. You do not need to say yes to everyone. This applies to your personal life, and to work. Do not agree to unreasonable deadlines because you want to influence your boss unless you are 100% sure you will be able to complete the task. If you've got a job, and you're not sure how to do it, do not be afraid to ask for help. If you work in a full-time job and have a family you care about, do not stick to your child's school. Know your limits! This applies to your time, energy, emotions, and skills. Modesty works side by side with honesty.

Chapter 3 do not lie to yourself

Lies make life difficult and often do not realize the far-reaching implications of their actions. Lying makes us unhappy people, who are constantly forced to cover our paths and watch our appearance. In fact, there are some poisonous things as a liar. We must never allow the negative in this world to force us to become dishonest people. It will put you lying near the door that leads to cheating and theft. Quit while you are advanced. Just think about the possible consequences of a single act of dishonesty. You must control yourself.

To be honest requires to be morally upright in everything. In other words, we will try to be honest in everything and gain trust around us, through our actions. Honesty is easy but to be honest requires you to effort. You can start gradually until you have mastered the art of honesty.

Man needs to cover his mistakes and hide them from others. So if you find yourself trying to hide some things from people try to avoid these actions or you will not be honest with yourself.

The benefits of integrity far outweigh any challenges that may be envisaged as a result of this session. Think of peace of mind not having to rethink every move or watch on your shoulder because you are always afraid of your discovery. Imagine that you woke up and were not burdened with heavy guilt as a result of your actions. Do not be fooled into thinking that no one is benefiting from your sincerity. It is very easy to be attracted to a respectful person. Most employers share quality as being of utmost importance when looking for new recruits or thinking about promoting someone within their organization.

To be honest does not mean that we must volunteer with all our secret affairs to anyone trying to benefit from our actions. Instead, we should not withhold relevant information from individuals who deserve an honest answer. To be honest does not also mean that the overbearing in things to get more than we deserve or make someone to believe something about ourselves is false. However, there are times when some of us may find honesty drive to catastrophic situations.

Honesty gives you happiness so if you find that lying gives you or give others happiness, then there is nothing wrong with it. It may be in three situations: to lie to your wife to improve the relationship between you, to lie to some friends to reunite them, to lie to someone who wants to deceive you.

Chapter 4 Improve your behavior

"Good behavior drive to good results"

To be good means to be warm, caring, gentle and friendly. To get a friend, you must be a friend. More vulgar words are "feather birds, gathering together." If you want to attract happy people and supporters to your life, you must be kind person. Why would anyone want to be around you otherwise?

People will remember what interaction you are doing and how it make them feel. When we are tough, we make life around us much more difficult than it should be. We make people feel unloved, feel we do not appreciate them, and they isolated when we want to be friends.

Do you want someone to treat you this way? Do you enjoy this cruel treatment? Do not you think that treating people this way at work, at school or at home, makes your life much harder than it should be? Kindness enhances the spirit of cooperation, even among people who do not really know each other. Engaging yourself in people who are ready to work next to you is much easier than trying to overcome this world on its own.

Our words are the most common forms of hardness. It can be interpreted as being harsh, arrogant, or even surprising as unpleasant. Using your words to put and elevate others is not only unpleasant, it is also a very selfish act, which often causes more harm than good. A major aspect of kindness is being courteous. Let's take some time to learn more about this beautiful quality.

Being polite is not as difficult as some think. While it is true that you're being polite is more difficult because of the negative attitudes of people around us, but it is not impossible. Being polite may magnify the ego of these individuals, but being polite is not in their hopes.

Being courteous reflects positively on our personality. Individuals are often seen as polite in terms of type, principles, professionalism and fun. With this very interdependent world in which we live, you never know who has insulted him.

Just imagine how embarrassing you are if you show up for a work interview, just to realize that the guy you've just cursed in the parking lot, because you think you've been stopped in your place, is actually the person being interviewed. Trust me, it has happened so many times before it can happen to you.

Being polite and gentle will make you very loved and will encourage others to share life with you. Another benefit of being polite is that will make it easy for you to get respect from those around you.

Even if they do not change their behavior immediately, they will have to respect you and your standards. In the end, they may change for the better as a result of your efforts. Would not life be easier if we all had jobs that our employees, subordinates and colleagues treated us with respect? Respect must be earned and polite should be one of the easiest ways to win.

I want to be courteous and gentle. If this is your decision you should follow some of these tips.

- Do not say anything that is not nice to others and do not publish it in social networking sites.

- Always smiling with others does not cost you anything, but it also makes you more and more handsome.

- Greet others when you see them, even if you do not know them.

- Do not detract from others' efforts. They may have done their best to please someone you might be.

- Encourage them and thank them even if you do not want what they do.

- Learn about the general culture of others so as not to offend them.

- Accept the opinion and opinion of others and do not be closed to yourself.

- Do not be stubborn in making the right decision just for you. Share decisions with others.

- Do not monopolize conversations by talking about yourself and your accomplishments.

- When someone comes to you. You have to give him full attention.

Chapter 5- the meaning of forgiving

"You must forgive others because it will come a day you need others to forgive you"

It is not easy to forgive. The mere need to use the word means that we have somehow been harmed. Grievance, whether real or imagined, will be one of the best gifts you can give yourself. This is whether you think the individual deserves such kindness or not. When we refuse to forgive, we become resentful. Clinging to the absurd is like drinking poison and expecting the person who hurt us will die. It can also be compared to causing injuries to our bodies, and we expect someone else to feel pain.

This logic is not only flawed, it is also very dangerous. Discontent can easily become hatred and hatred is something very ugly. But why do we find it difficult to tolerate? If pardoning someone who harms us is going to benefit, why should the idea of giving up harm make us uncomfortable?

The real problem lies in the fact that none of us wants to continue to terrorize any mistake we have had. But as we continue to think about the extent of the damage done to us, we unconsciously began to think about making the individual pay for what they did. Our shameful sense of justice often compels us to believe that if we retain all the pain that has caused us and refuse to let him go, we will have the justice we deserve.

This is especially true when the individual does not appear to be sorry for what they have done. Unfortunately, we cannot force an individual to become a better person by withholding his or her property from them. We only hurt ourselves and we force our minds to ease the pain again and again.

While we are very angry at life with the weight of discontent in our hearts, our speech, and our mood will be negatively affected.

Despite the fact that we may have been wrong with an individual or perhaps some individuals, everyone around us will begin to be affected. Discontent often makes us nervous, depressed, and not happy in general. To make matters worse, it is often the people we love and not the people who hurt us, who will suffer as a result of what happened.

It is also known that the discontent affects our memory, productivity at work, ability to perform routine tasks, ability to focus, and even sex drive. The bitterness and rejection of forgiveness are also associated with weak immune system, poor heart condition and even high blood pressure. As you can see, rejecting forgiveness will never be helpful.

But what exactly is forgiveness? Is it simply forgetting what happened? Does forgiveness mean that we simply pretend that nothing happened? Both. It's not that simple. When we forgive, we must involve more than our words. We must change our way of thinking and feeling towards the individual. It looks like we're letting them start a clean page again. You refuse to allow the situation to cause you or the parties involved to harm you for longer. This requires a high level of emotional intelligence, restraint, and love. Forgiveness is not simply "free of punishment" for what they have done, but it allows participants to stop dwelling in the past and move on to more important things.

"Forgiveness means that you fill yourself with love, and you radiate that love outward. You need to refuse to hang onto the venom or hatred that was

engendered by the behaviors that caused the wounds." - Wayne Dyer

Your anger is the result of someone else's actions, and allowing yourself to continue because of what happened for an extended period of time, is to really give the person your keys to your happiness. It seems as though you are allowing this person to control you, and will continue to control you until you have gathered the courage to forgive you.

Forgiveness is also useful because it often results when we know our own mistakes. It becomes easier for us to forgive when we remember that we have to ask forgiveness many times. Contrary to what we believe, we are not perfect. We sometimes hurt people around us, even those we love, without realizing it. When we refuse to harbor resentment and practice forgiveness, it will be easy for those around us to forgive us when we sin.

Here are some of the reasons why it is useful to practice forgiveness:

- You will be happier and in a much better mood.
- You will sleep better at night.
- You will not jeopardize your business.
- Your relationship with other important people or your family will not be compromised.
- You will learn more self-control and self-awareness.
- You will enjoy more peace.
- You will gain respect from those around you.
- You will no longer feel the pain of the damage.
- You will suffer from less anxiety.
- You will become more respectful of yourself while observing your own strength.

Being tolerant does not mean you have to be motivated and allow yourself to be hurt again and again. While you will leave any complaint you may have against the party or parties that have offended you, then you certainly do not have to put yourself in a position to be hurt in this way again. It is perfectly acceptable to be more careful now that you have seen what these people can do. But, please be very careful. In the case of minor offenses, which are not intentionally malicious, do not make a mistake assuming that the act represents the person concerned. Please remember that we all make mistakes, and we also caused another pain.

Forgiveness is also not an opportunity for revenge. Declaring that you have forgiven someone is not an ad that you have the "upper hand". The people concerned may be guilty, but they certainly do not owe you anything. Even if they did not apologize, they gained a lot by expanding this offer for peace, and dispensing with the bitterness that was consumed one day. Remember that through tolerance, you are doing your own well-known. While they may benefit as a result of your decision, their exemption is actually a gift for yourself.

Because we both realize that forgiving someone hurts you is not easy, I will never ask you to do it immediately or all at once. You have the option of tolerance in stages. Gradually forgiving people who have sinned, will ensure you have time to eradicate any bitterness you have towards them, from your mind and heart. If you get a chance to see this person often, you can start with the word hello.

This may be a surprise to them because they do not expect such a generous gesture, and that may open the way for the discussion that both of them need to close for some time. Sometimes, even though you have been wronged, it is best to take the initiative to put things right. Always remember how this modest work will benefit you in the long term, whether they appreciate this gesture or not.

Another simple exercise that helps us to forgive is to write down the name of the person or people who annoy you and list everything they have done to bother you. Once you have completed that list, write down a list of all the events that have hurt someone else and ask forgiveness from them. This is not something we tend to think about. We see in black and white how many times we have allowed our bad habits to hurt those around us, especially those we love, it may be just the payment we need to give up any grudges we may have. What is most disturbing for some individuals is when they see the names of the person they have resented on the list of people who had to ask for forgiveness.

Other useful exercises provide a list of all the good things that this person has done for you. This exercise will help you remember that despite their mistakes, this individual or these individuals also have many beautiful qualities. In the case of those closest to us, these qualities are why we loved them and kept them close in the first place. You will make the world a better place by helping just one individual to become a better person. Such kindness does not pass unnoticed or without reward.

Take a very strong person to be tolerant. But think of how much better than our lives if we do not wander with bitterness every day. Leaving this heavy burden is one of the best ways to heal ourselves. This world has already been a disaster, and it definitely does not need more discontent to

make it worse.

Chapter 6-give to love

Do not ask the generous person to give all his belongings. The generous person is also not required to allow others to pay them. Being generous involves first the willingness to offer or the desire to give more than is required. Being generous takes kindness to the next level. You may be nice at heart and often think of helping others, but if you do not actually take the time to help someone else, then you have not really mastered the art of being generous. Our generosity prompts us to give ourselves willingly, and expect nothing in return.

I know you should be wondering how giving up your assets can help you live a better life. The truth is that many often consider generosity as one of the keys to true happiness in this miserable world. In fact, many medical practitioners testify to the fact that being generous is also very good for your health. Often a generous person looks for opportunities to do good for others. Just think of the volunteers who make their way to help Soup Kitchens at the end of each week. Those of us brave enough to register in the Peace Corps are also considered very generous. But just help the old lady with grocery bags, or stop to let the child cross the road, can be considered generous. This kind of interest to others proves to be useful because it compels us to focus on the needs of others rather than our own problems. Anything that minimizes the impact of our problems, whether in our relationships or even financially, will have a direct impact on our health. It preserves our generosity to protect us from all the irony and narcissism that make it very difficult to navigate through this world.

However, I would encourage you to be careful while your steps to be more generous. Be very careful how you demonstrate your generosity. Please be especially careful when you are generous to members of the opposite sex. If you have already taken it, do not want to send the wrong impression, avoid personalized gifts or gifts. A personal gift is anything related to one's body. Perfumes, for example, will be considered a personal gift.

Please also bear in mind that your own safety may play its role when it is gracious. Many people were robbed when a homeless person asked them to make some money. Getting to your wallet or bag, checking where your money is and how much money you have, is a bad idea, no matter how much you need it. The safest option would be to tell the person that you will return with a gift.

I strongly suggest that you go to a safe place, away from prying eyes, and pack everything you would like to donate to that person in advance. My last word of caution is that you need to feel the person before you are too generous. Some people prefer spontaneity and others prefer if you ask them first if they need your help. Even the best intentions can put you in embarrassing situations if they are not implemented correctly.

Chapter 7-be yourself

We all need to learn to be ourselves again. This is one of the most important aspects of successfully navigating through this disaster that we call life. This encouragement does not give you the right to be joking. We have already discussed that healing ourselves from the pain of this world requires us to work hard to get rid of our negative qualities.

Attributes like being arrogant, rude, dishonest and stealth have no place in your life. When we roam proudly with these ugly habits, we call all kinds of negativity in our lives. The result is more pain and disappointment. That's why I encouraged you in chapter one to get to know yourself. This will equip you better to heal yourself, by learning more about your mistakes. What exactly does it mean to be yourself? It requires you to distance yourself from all the signs imposed on us by the world around us. These ugly posters come because of the way we look at them, the way we wear them, or even the society in which we grew up. There is no reason why we allow the world around us to press us into a mold that does not truly represent who we are. Just thinking about how to edit it will not have to pretend to be something you are not. That's all I can of course. We will never want to take some liberties that may have far-reaching effects on our personal lives and may even jeopardize our jobs. This means that you may want to stick to anything radical, such as your hair dying purple and green, until you find the employer who wishes to accommodate this choice.

Here are 5 important reasons you need to start to correct yourself:

1. You will not be able to satisfy everyone. If you always allow people around you to identify yourself, you'll always have to change what you're

trying to make everyone happy. The only problem with this is that you will deal with many conflicting demands that will end up being a disappointing person. In addition, putting yourself under this kind of pressure will make you feel dissatisfied in the end.

2. The community around us does not know what it wants. The media portray both the housewife and the wicked businessman as the ideal woman. The community also demands that men be sensitive to the needs of the opposite sex and bad boys as well. What would you be if you simply let those around you determine who you are? No matter what you decide to be, just remember that it is very stressful to put this kind of offer every day.

3. You will end up making life-changing decisions based on the whims of people around you who will not suffer the consequences of these choices.

If you decide to have a child, just because your family thinks it is time, you will be the one who should take care of that child! If you decide to pursue your career because your peers think you will do a good job there, you will have to live with the burden of a career you hate forever.

4. The truth always appears. Sooner or later, people will begin to realize that you are forging. Unfortunately, as we see in the case of many celebrities, the truth often comes in a scandal or a major collapse.

5. When you are satisfied with your identity, you will be really happy. How can you love yourself, when you constantly pretend that you are something you are not?

When told and doing everything, you need to control your life if you want to see real improvements. You cannot expect different results if you are not bold enough to make radical changes. The time for these changes is now!

In the end I hope you know that healing the soul comes through feeling some happiness. This life does not deserve to be miserable. Forget the past and live in the present.